T0225233

Cambridge Elements ≡

Elements of Improving Quality and Safety in Healthcare
edited by
Mary Dixon-Woods,* Katrina Brown,* Sonja Marjanovic,†
Tom Ling,† Ellen Perry,* and Graham Martin*
*THIS Institute (The Healthcare Improvement Studies Institute)
†RAND Europe

HEALTH ECONOMICS

Andrew Street[1] and Nils Gutacker[2]

[1] Department of Health Policy, London School of Economics and Political Science
[2] Centre for Health Economics, University of York

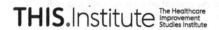
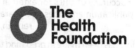

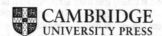

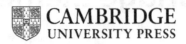

CAMBRIDGE
UNIVERSITY PRESS

Shaftesbury Road, Cambridge CB2 8EA, United Kingdom

One Liberty Plaza, 20th Floor, New York, NY 10006, USA

477 Williamstown Road, Port Melbourne, VIC 3207, Australia

314–321, 3rd Floor, Plot 3, Splendor Forum, Jasola District Centre,
New Delhi – 110025, India

103 Penang Road, #05–06/07, Visioncrest Commercial, Singapore 238467

Cambridge University Press is part of Cambridge University Press & Assessment,
a department of the University of Cambridge.

We share the University's mission to contribute to society through the pursuit of
education, learning and research at the highest international levels of excellence.

www.cambridge.org
Information on this title: www.cambridge.org/9781009454209

DOI: 10.1017/9781009325974

First published 2023

A catalogue record for this publication is available from the British Library.

ISBN 978-1-009-45420-9 Hardback
ISBN 978-1-009-32598-1 Paperback
ISSN 2754-2912 (online)
ISSN 2754-2904 (print)

Health Economics

Elements of Improving Quality and Safety in Healthcare

DOI: 10.1017/9781009325974
First published online: December 2023

Andrew Street[1] and Nils Gutacker[2]

[1]*Department of Health Policy, London School of Economics and Political Science*

[2]*Centre for Health Economics, University of York*

Author for correspondence: Andrew Street, a.street@lse.ac.uk

Abstract: This Element examines economic perspectives on improving quality and safety in healthcare. Though competition is generally recognised by economists as an important driver of improvement, it may not work so straightforwardly in healthcare – in part because some services are provided by very few organisations, but also because people are not always easily able to judge healthcare quality and rarely have to pay the full price for services. Different approaches for stimulating improvement are therefore needed, and the authors look at examples from the care home, primary care, and hospital sectors. They emphasise the need for economic evaluation of improvement efforts, based on the principle that improvement activities should only be undertaken if the benefits are worth at least the costs of implementing and running them. Using examples, they explain the economic approach to evaluating how benefits and costs of improvement efforts can be compared by applying cost-effectiveness analysis. This title is also available as Open Access on Cambridge Core.

Keywords: value for money, competition, incentives, economic evaluation, cost-effectiveness analysis

ISBNs: 9781009454209 (HB), 9781009325981 (PB), 9781009325974 (OC)
ISSNs: 2754-2912 (online), 2754-2904 (print)

Contents

1 Introduction

Over the past few decades, economics has gained prominence in many areas of public policy. Though once it focused predominantly on issues such as employment, inflation, and taxation, the reach of economics now extends to a wide range of areas, such as social security, education, and the environment. Healthcare is no exception to this trend. Governmental bodies the world over now seek economic expertise and advice on the regulation, financing, and provision of healthcare.

Economics is perhaps best described as a way of seeing the world rather than a particular methodology for improving healthcare; so it is important that those who work in the healthcare system understand how economists view the world and seek to shape it. As a discipline, health economics covers a wide scope of topics, as set out in the textbook by Morris et al.[1]

In this Element, we will primarily focus on two important issues: economic perspectives on *stimulating* improvement and the role of economic evaluation in *evaluating* healthcare improvement activities. Our overall aim is to provide readers with an intuitive understanding of the value of economic thinking in healthcare improvement and to facilitate critical thinking in this area. We offer a particular, though not exclusive, focus on the English National Health Service (NHS).

2 The Economic Approach to Healthcare Improvement

We start with a brief introduction to the economic approach to improving healthcare. All governments play a key role in shaping their country's healthcare system through some combination of regulation, financing, and provision of healthcare. In the UK, the four constituent governments determine a large share of the amount of money that is available for spending on healthcare. Invariably, the amount available falls short of demand.[2] The difference between demand and the amount of care that can be delivered within limited resources means that trade-offs are inevitable, and difficult choices have to be made.

One common challenge arises because of what are called 'opportunity costs'. Every time we use resources for one purpose, we give up the opportunity to use them for something else that may also be beneficial. Examples of areas where opportunity costs are sometimes considered too high include very expensive cancer drugs[3] and cosmetic surgery.[4] All of these things may have intrinsic value, but the health benefits they generate may be smaller than the health benefits that would have to be sacrificed elsewhere to fund them. Policymakers may therefore decide that the limited funds available would be better spent in other ways.

2.1 Seeking Value for Money

UK governments face frequent calls to increase the amount of money they spend on healthcare. But to heed these calls, governments have to find the money from somewhere, whether by cutting expenses on other government-funded services (e.g. welfare, policing, etc.) or raising taxes. An alternative is to encourage the healthcare system to make better use of the resources it already has, so that same overall budget could deliver better value. It might be possible, for example, to reduce the resources needed to provide services by cutting wasteful spending[5] or through innovations, service improvements, or new technologies. Such efforts might, for instance, include switching from branded to generic drugs,[6] reusing medical devices,[7] or changing the skill mix of the healthcare workers who deliver the service.[8] These kinds of changes might be able to yield savings that could be reinvested in the healthcare system.

But can healthcare services be both motivated to and, in fact, improve care to make it better or cheaper? In most sectors of the economy, the pressure to improve lies in a well-functioning market; so competition is the main driver. If a well-functioning market does not exist, economists often propose system-level policies that seek to emulate the effect of competitive pressures. These often take the form of changes in funding or regulation of services. This is the key and distinctive economic approach to healthcare improvement.

2.2 Competition as a Spur to Improvement

Now, we first consider what a well-functioning market would look like before turning to a discussion of market imperfections. We then review some factors that explain why well-functioning markets are unlikely to arise in healthcare.

Economists see competition as driving organisations to improve and innovate – potentially yielding benefits to consumers and service users in the form of lower prices, higher quality, or a combination of both. *Perfect* competition arises when consumers are fully aware of the quality of the goods or services they are buying, that the goods or services provided by different organisations are pretty much identical (or readily comparable), and that organisations cannot charge a higher price than the going market rate.

In these circumstances, organisations have to work hard to attract customers. That means keeping up with their competitors. For example, if an organisation introduces a technological improvement that allows it to reduce prices or improve quality, it has a chance to attract new customers and sell more products. But other organisations may quickly adopt the new technology and follow suit in order to retain their own market share – so the benefits are quickly passed on to all consumers in the form of price reductions or quality improvements.

Any organisation that fails to react risks losing customers or going out of business altogether. In this cut-throat context, organisations either 'innovate or die'.[9]

The opposite extreme to perfect competition is a world dominated by monopolists, which are the sole and exclusive providers of particular goods or services. For example, monopolists have been or still are responsible for the provision of water, electricity, railways, or postal services in most countries. Facing no competition, monopolists have little incentive to innovate or make improvements. If customers think they are being charged too much or are unhappy with the quality of a product or service, they cannot shop around for a better option since nothing else is on offer. Customers then face a stark choice: take it or leave it. This can make monopolists complacent. Their only incentive is to make the minimum improvements needed to discourage potential competitors from entering the market.

Unsurprisingly, monopolists may put more effort into protecting their monopoly power than into seeking technological improvements. Monopoly power can be used to earn large profits: facing no competition, they can charge what they like and keep prices high. This is bad for consumers, who have to pay higher prices for lower quality goods and services than they would if there was more than one supplier that they could go to. Competition (or antitrust) law is designed to prevent the creation of monopolies and limit the abuse of monopoly power.

Healthcare can feature different types of competitive environments. Table 1 shows three English examples, which will be considered in more detail in Section 3. Some organisations – such as an isolated hospital serving a rural community – might be regarded as local monopolists. Other parts of the health and social care system may have more competitive characteristics since they feature a great many organisations, such as care homes or general practice, providing similar types of service. Yet, even though we might expect competitive pressure to be greater in these settings, it might not ensure high-quality, affordable healthcare. This is because two important and distinctive features reduce the competitive imperatives that healthcare organisations face: first, it is often difficult to assess quality, and, second, people are often protected from bearing the full cost of services.

2.2.1 Quality Is Hard to Assess

Another distinctive feature of healthcare is that the quality of healthcare services is often very difficult to assess before, during, and after treatment. This means that a key requirement for perfect competition is not met because people are rarely well-placed to act as well-informed consumers in relation to healthcare.

Table 1 A comparison of selected health and care sectors in England

Sector	Example product or service	Number of competitors	Price awareness	Quality awareness	Example of approach to reduce cost or price	Example of approach to improve quality
Care homes	Residential care for dementia patients	Many	High: most individuals pay full price	Difficult to assess for residents and their families	Competition	CQC inspections[10]
GP practices	Range of primary care services	Some in local area	Zero: consumers pay nothing at point of use	Reasonably high, especially for regular attenders	GP contract negotiated between government and BMA[11]	Quality and Outcomes Framework[12]
Hospitals	Range of elective, emergency, A&E, and outpatient services	Local monopoly	Zero: consumers pay nothing at point of use	Medium: publicly reported data	National tariff payment system for hospital services[13]	CQC inspections; public reporting

CQC = Care Quality Commission. A&E = accident and emergency. BMA = British Medical Association.

Sometimes people have difficulty assessing their need for care,[14] notably when health problems are undetected (e.g. an undiagnosed cancer). Even if people are aware that they have a problem, they may lack the expertise to know what to do or how to do it. This is why they are so reliant on medical experts such as general practitioners (GPs) to provide them with diagnostic information and advice about treatment options. Economists describe this as a 'principal–agent' relationship.[15,16] Reliance on experts is not unique to healthcare: people commonly rely on mechanics or plumbers to service their vehicles or heating systems and to diagnose any faults that need to be rectified. But the extent to which people seek expert advice is often more pronounced in healthcare than in other areas of economic activity. Occasionally, this can lead to abuse. For example, Dr Ian Paterson inflicted medically unjustified procedures on women who had found a lump in their breast but were not in a position to determine what care was needed.[17] But even when doctors act in the best interests of their patients, people can find it difficult to judge whether the healthcare services they received were of the highest possible quality.

One of the key reasons that make it hard to judge the quality of services is that there is an unclear relationship between the treatment received and the outcome for an individual patient. If someone recovers, was this the result of treatment or would they have recovered anyway? Why do some people enjoy higher post-treatment health status than others? And why do some people suffer poorer post-treatment health status – or even death? These challenges in determining whether a treatment *worked* and the influences on the outcome make it very difficult to assess the quality and value of healthcare – even for members of the medical profession themselves.

Overall, because patients or would-be patients do not always share the characteristics of well-informed customers, competition in the usual sense is not straightforward for healthcare.

2.2.2 Financial Protection at Point of Use

A further distinctive feature of the healthcare sector, at least in many high-income and middle-income countries, is that people are often protected against the full cost of healthcare services. This means that they may pay little, if any, attention to prices when making decisions about what services to use or who to buy from. This in turn means healthcare organisations face little direct pressure from service users to reduce their costs.

The extent to which people enjoy financial protection from healthcare expenses varies from country to country and across services. Many countries fund their healthcare systems either from taxation or via some form of health insurance. In tax-based systems, most services are free at the point of use, although there might be co-payments for some services, such as pharmaceutical prescriptions (England, Norway, and Spain) or GP visits (Australia, New Zealand, Norway, and Sweden).[18] In countries with insurance-based systems, such as Germany, France, and the USA, people usually have to make a contribution towards the cost of the services they receive, perhaps in the form of insurance premiums, co-payments, or deductibles; they rarely have to pay the full amount.

The more that people have to pay for services themselves, the more likely they are to shop around for the lowest price or best-value services. By contrast, when people have to pay nothing at all for a service, individual consumers might have very little, if any, knowledge of its price or cost and so may exercise very little cost control over healthcare providers. This gives rise to a problem: potentially, providers could charge what they like and pass the costs on to taxpayers under a tax-based system or on to insurers under an insurance-based system. But the money has to come from somewhere, either in the form of higher tax or insurance contributions or by cutting healthcare expenditure elsewhere in the system. Thus, there is a trade-off: the downside of financial protection for individuals is that healthcare providers are under less pressure to reduce their costs.

3 Stimulating Healthcare Improvement

Three important ideas guide the types of activities that economists have proposed to stimulate and encourage healthcare improvement. First, economists think about improvements in healthcare as having the potential to yield two forms of benefit: higher quality and/or lower cost. Quality can be defined as anything that people value from a service, such as better health-related quality of life (HRQoL), satisfaction with how the service is delivered, higher safety, or provision of care according to the best clinical practice. Lower costs can mean cost savings, which can be reinvested to pay for more or better healthcare. Second, economists are interested in the environment in which organisations operate because it influences both the incentives for organisations to make improvements and the likelihood that cost reductions are reinvested. Third, as we noted earlier, economists also recognise that healthcare systems are distinctive and different from other parts of the economy, most notably because people may not always be able to assess the quality of care accurately and are insulated (perhaps completely) from having to pay for care.

When organisations face little competitive pressure, when quality is hard to assess, and when service users pay limited attention to costs or prices, economists say that 'market failure' can occur. The risk is that innovations and improvements then emerge and spread more slowly than they would in more competitive environments. In order to speed up improvement and ensure an appropriate balance between efforts to reduce costs and improve quality, economists may advocate fostering greater competition or using other approaches to put pressure on healthcare organisations to make improvements. In this section, we look at how this plays out in three examples of healthcare and social care sectors in the UK, starting with a sector that has many service providers (care homes – Section 3.1) and then considering sectors with progressively fewer organisations (primary care – Section 3.2, and hospitals – Section 3.3). For each, we assess the strength of competitive forces and the form of interventions that have been developed to foster cost control and stimulate improvement.

3.1 Care Homes

As populations become progressively older, the care home sector is assuming greater responsibility for providing round-the-clock care for older people who can no longer live independently. Residential care homes cater for people who need help with their personal care, such as washing and dressing. Nursing homes support people who have health conditions that require support from qualified nursing staff. The majority (80%) of the 11,000 care homes in the UK are run by private, for-profit organisations, while the remaining fifth are run by voluntary or charitable organisations or by local authorities on a not-for-profit basis.[19] Around 4,000 (36%) are standalone care homes; the rest are run as part of groups. The largest six chains own more than 100 care homes each and together account for 11% of the total number of homes.

Simply by virtue of the large number of care homes, the sector has the potential to be quite competitive. But users of care homes (or their family members) are also very price-conscious. Moving to a care home is a major and expensive decision. In England, nursing home care for someone with dementia costs over £800 a week, usually payable for the rest of that individual's life.[20] Financial support varies across the constituent countries of the UK. England is the least generous, in 2023 providing up to £92.40 a week (as an Attendance Allowance) towards the costs, but no other financial support until the individual's assets fall below £23,250.[21]

Because of the large number of care homes and people's sensitivity to price, there is considerable price competition in the English care home sector.[22] The result is that care homes typically earn just enough to cover costs, with many care homes struggling to break even.[23] There is evidence that care homes may seek to compromise on quality in an attempt to keep costs low;[22] yet, they may be exposed to limited challenge from 'customers' themselves because many service users, such as those with dementia, may not be able to assess or influence the quality of care. This makes service users vulnerable to poor quality care and worse, with more than 67,500 allegations of abuse in care homes in 2018.[24]

Given that individuals are in such a vulnerable position, the care home sector is highly regulated. In England, care homes need to be registered by the Care Quality Commission, which conducts regular inspections to ensure that ' . . . the service is safe, effective, caring, responsive and well-led'.[10] If inadequacies are found, the frequency of inspections increases and care homes are required to make improvements as specified in the Care Quality Commission's inspection report. Care homes are also required to provide a summary of and a link to the most recent inspection report on their website.

In summary, the care home sector features many providers competing for custom by keeping costs and prices low. But because users struggle to assess quality and have limited power to influence it, providers may respond to price competition by cutting their costs in ways that have implications for their ability to deliver safe, respectful care. Economists would support initiatives to improve quality measurement and reporting so that service users can make more informed decisions. But it may also be necessary for regulators to set and enforce quality standards to protect vulnerable service users.

3.2 Primary Care

Like the care home sector, the primary care sector is characterised by a large number of relatively small providers. In England, for instance, there are about 7,000 GP practices, each serving an average of 9,000 patients.[25] But unlike the care home sector, patients do not pay directly for the services they receive. This means they are not typically price-conscious, as they do not need to worry about the cost of services when deciding whether and where to seek primary care. As a result, GPs face no direct pressure from patients to keep their costs down; that pressure has to come from elsewhere.

Patients might, of course, be sensitive to quality in their choices relating to primary care, but the evidence suggests that they take little account of quality when deciding which practice to register with.[26,27] And once registered, people tend to stay with the same practice, switching only if they move to a different neighbourhood.[28] Loyalty is particularly evident among patients with chronic conditions, who may build long-term personal relationships with their GPs.[29] Attempts have been made over the years both to make it easier for people to change practice and to encourage GPs to compete for those patients. This was the key aim of the general practice fundholding scheme advocated by Maynard, a health economist, in the 1980s and implemented by the Conservative government in 1989.[30,31] The idea was that if it was easier for patients to change practice, GPs would improve the quality of primary care services to attract new patients. Although some evidence suggests that the scheme did improve quality, the benefits did not justify the costs.[32] Since then, efforts have been made to make it even easier for patients to switch GP practices, but it is clear that this, on its own, is not sufficient to drive improvement in primary care because very few people are actually prepared to change practices on a regular basis.[27]

Since patients do not pay for primary care and only rarely shop around to choose their practice, the standard competitive mechanisms to encourage cost control and improve quality in primary care are weak. Instead, more recent UK policy has relied on the system by which GPs are paid to achieve these two objectives. Traditionally, though not exclusively, GPs in the UK are paid via a mixture of capitation, fee-for-service, and specific payments reflecting local circumstances, such as rurality and staff costs.[11] These forms of payment allow the government to control costs, but they do not encourage improvement explicitly. To address this, the UK introduced a pay-for-performance scheme for GPs known as the Quality and Outcomes Framework (QOF; see Box 1).

The QOF awards extra payments to GPs who deliver high-quality care according to pre-specified definitions of quality. GPs who invest in quality are able to earn more money, allowing them to recoup the costs of investment and, possibly, generate a surplus. GPs who do not improve quality on the chosen measures are likely to lose out financially. Evidence suggests that the QOF has helped improve the quality of primary care services – but only for those things for which payments are made. Research has also identified the risk that GPs could become alienated by pay-for-performance schemes that are perceived to remove some of their clinical autonomy and encourage 'box ticking'.[38]

In summary, despite the large number of general practices in the UK, competitive pressure on GPs to reduce costs or improve quality is weak. This is because patients are not price-conscious, as they do not have to pay for care, and patients rarely switch their practice because of poor quality. So the government relies on payments to GPs as the predominant means to encourage them to improve quality as well as to control costs.

3.3 Hospital Market

In most countries, the majority of hospitals face little competition, sometimes by design. In England, for example, plans were implemented from the 1960s to create district general hospitals to serve the needs of their geographically

BOX 1 THE QUALITY AND OUTCOMES FRAMEWORK

Introduced in April 2004, the QOF seeks to improve population health by incentivising GPs to deliver lifestyle interventions such as smoking cessation and to meet specific quality targets in the management of common chronic conditions, such as heart disease, diabetes, and asthma.[12] Although voluntary, the QOF covers nearly all GP practices and so applies to the vast majority of the population. The total QOF expenditure in England in 2020–21 was approximately £700 million per year or 8% of average practice income, which makes it economically significant.[33]

Did the introduction of the QOF lead to improvements in primary care? Yes and no. Its introduction was associated with rapid improvements in targeted activities, but these improvements were typically modest in size and accompanied by some unintended negative impacts on non-incentivised activities.[34] Disparities in the provision of incentivised activities diminished under the QOF, as poorer-performing practices in more deprived areas improved at fastest rates.[35] This was likely due to increasing payments being awarded for increasing achievement, so that practices with lower baseline performance had a greater incentive to improve.

It is less clear whether the QOF led to improvements in population health. There is some evidence that emergency hospital admissions fell for some conditions with incentivised activities, such as coronary heart disease, but not others.[36] There are also indications that the QOF may have reduced mortality for incentivised conditions, although the findings are not statistically significant by usual standards.[37] Overall, this suggests that pay-for-performance can help induce some improvement effort in primary care, but this effort translates into better health only with careful design of the incentives.

defined catchment populations of around 100,000–150,000.[39] Subsequent consolidation means that, in 2023, there were around 135 acute hospitals located across England, such that most people have a local hospital reasonably nearby. As a consequence, the NHS hospital sector comprises a set of local monopoly hospitals, each serving a defined population.

Patients in the UK do not have to pay directly towards the cost of their hospital care; so they do not need to worry about the direct financial consequences of receiving treatment. The advantage of this arrangement is that access to hospital care is (in principle at least) equitable both in geographical and financial terms because access does not depend on where people live or how much they can afford to pay. The disadvantage is that hospitals might face little pressure to manage their costs or quality; they are not competing for patients with other hospitals in the vicinity, and patients are not price-conscious.

The government has tried to encourage cost control by acting as a monopsonist (or sole) purchaser of hospital services. This means that the government sets the prices according to which hospitals are paid under a system called 'yardstick competition', which has become the dominant form of hospital reimbursement in most European countries.[40] Under this system, all English hospitals are paid the same price (the national tariff) for treating a patient of a particular type, defined using what are called Healthcare Resource Groups.[41] The price is based on costs reported by all English hospitals – so each hospital has minimal influence on the price it receives for doing a procedure or other intervention. By translating this cost information into prices, the government is, in effect, making hospitals compete with each other to reduce their costs, with lower-cost hospitals providing a yardstick that other higher-cost hospitals should aspire to. Evidence from around the world suggests that the introduction of yardstick competition has been associated with reductions in length of stay and a slowdown in the rate of growth of healthcare spending.[42]

As with care homes, the risk of encouraging hospitals to reduce their costs is that they might do so by reducing quality. So in addition to regulation through the Care Quality Commission, which operates an inspection regime, economists have lent their support to two other general approaches to guard against hospitals responding in this undesirable way.

The first is to make available more information about the quality of care, either so that hospitals are 'named and shamed' into addressing shortcomings or so that patients can make more informed decisions about where to seek care, perhaps bypassing their local hospital. The NHS is at the forefront internationally in making detailed comparative information available in an accessible fashion to the general public. For example, since 2014, the NHS has published comparative data on the performance of surgeons.[43] But there are questions about whether patients actually access or act on such information. For example, the MyNHS website, which made a range of comparative health and care data available in one place, was decommissioned because not enough people used it.[44]

The second approach has been to reward or penalise hospitals according to the quality of care they provided. In the past, these arrangements were non-financial. An example was the so-called 'targets and terror' regime under which hospital chief executives faced the sack if patients were not treated within a specified timeframe.[45] Since 2010, the English government has attached financial rewards or penalties to quality by implementing pay-for-performance arrangements, notably in the form of Best Practice Tariffs. These are designed to encourage hospitals to adopt best practice in providing care and to reimburse them for the costs of doing so.[46]

In other jurisdictions, hospitals are penalised for providing substandard care. In the USA, for example, fines are levied on hospitals with higher than expected emergency readmission rates for acute myocardial infarction, heart failure, and pneumonia.[47] Pay-for-performance schemes have been adopted in healthcare systems the world over and take a rich variety of forms, as masterfully detailed by Milstein and Schreyoegg.[48]

In summary, then, with hospitals facing limited competitive pressure, yardstick competition has been used to control hospital costs while inspection, public reporting, and financial incentives have all been used to encourage hospitals to improve quality.

4 Evaluating Healthcare Improvement Activities

In addition to their analyses of the incentives for innovation and improvement in healthcare organisations, economists have also established an evaluative approach to help decision-makers to determine which improvement activities offer value for money and whether they should be adopted. In this section, we briefly describe this approach, known as economic evaluation. Readers are referred to the excellent textbooks by Drummond et al.[49,50] for a more in-depth discussion.

4.1 The Evaluative Approach

Economists argue that resources should be deployed so that they yield the largest benefit in order to maximise social welfare – this is termed 'allocative efficiency'. In the context of the English NHS, allocative efficiency is commonly assumed to mean using the available healthcare budget to achieve the highest level of population health, although other important outcomes, such as patient experience, are also sometimes considered.[51]

There is no shortage of possible activities, programmes, interventions, and other efforts that could be undertaken with the aim of improving care. But many require additional resources. Those resources are not usually sitting idle, so they cannot be repurposed without giving up some other activity. This raises two questions: which improvement activities are worth adopting, and how can decision-makers ensure ' ... that the value of what is gained from an activity outweighs the value of what has to be sacrificed'?[52]

Cost-effectiveness analysis (CEA) is one of the most commonly used methods of economic evaluation to address these questions. CEA compares the incremental costs and benefits of two alternative courses of action: (1) the new improvement activity and (2) the current status quo being maintained.

Costs and benefits that are unaffected by the activity – that is, those that would occur in equal measure under both courses of action – can be ignored when conducting CEA.

Incremental costs are calculated by multiplying the additional amounts of healthcare resources that will be used as a result of the activity (e.g. implementing a protocol that requires additional staff) by their price (e.g. wages). Any resources that are indirectly used as a consequence of the activity should also be considered. For example, if the improvement activity means patients live longer, they may consume more healthcare services than would otherwise have been the case.

Incremental benefits can take various forms: for example, the benefit of an improvement activity can be measured in terms of clinical parameters (e.g. reduction in blood pressure[53] or blood glucose levels[54]), process improvements (e.g. reduction in waiting times[55]), behaviours (e.g. reduction in the number of safety incidents[56]), or changes in patient outcomes and time in hospital (e.g. reductions in mortality and length of stay[57]). In some evaluations, benefits beyond health impacts are considered.[58] In others, there may be 'positive externalities' with benefits extending beyond the immediate recipient to include family members or carers, for example.[59,60]

Many applications of CEA in economic evaluations in healthcare summarise incremental benefits in the form of quality-adjusted life years (QALYs), which combine the effect of an activity on life expectancy and HRQoL into a single number (see Box 2).[65] Using a common metric, such as the QALY, is useful because it allows comparisons across different disease groups and clinical settings.

In making these cost and benefit calculations, it is important to recognise that there may be upfront costs as well as long-term benefits. Some improvement activities may require investments before the first patient is treated (e.g. to change a building to adapt it for use by people who are disabled). Sometimes, the benefits of the activity may accrue long after it starts – for example, improvements in detecting hypertension may not show up as improvements in the health of patients for a long time.

To date, QALYs have not been used so much in economic evaluations in improvement activities, in part because many of these activities target processes that may not *directly* affect quality or length of life and in part because data linking improvement efforts to outcomes may not be easy to access or the causal chains may be hard to establish. In addition, the full long-term consequences of improvement activities are rarely measured as part of randomised trials or observational studies (see the Element on measurement for improvement[66]). Economists have therefore developed special statistical techniques, known as decision-analytical modelling, to extrapolate the total incremental costs and

Box 2 Calculating quality-adjusted life years

Economists have promoted the QALY as a composite measure of health that combines aspects of quality and quantity of life.[61-63] Quantity of life is given by the remaining number of years a patient can expect to live, which is often inferred by combining data on short-term survival (e.g. within 30 days of the intervention of interest) with long-term life expectancy estimates from actuary life tables. Evidence on HRQoL is typically measured via multi-attribute utility instruments, such as the EQ-5D, SF-6D, or HUI 3, which are scored so that a value of 1 denotes full HRQoL and 0 is equivalent to being dead.[64]

A patient's QALYs are calculated as the sum of life years weighed by the HRQoL experienced. A year in full health (i.e. HRQoL = 1) is equivalent to 1 QALY. A year spent in less than full health, for example due to pain or impaired mobility, is equivalent to <1 QALY, with the reduction being proportional to shortfall on the HRQoL scale.

Figure 1 demonstrates the calculation of QALYs for a hypothetical patient who underwent some healthcare intervention at the start of a clinical trial and then experienced two years of full HRQoL, three years of 0.4 HRQoL, and six months of 0.1 HRQoL before dying. By multiplying each duration with their HRQoL weight and summing across, we find that the patient enjoyed $(2 \times 1) + (3 \times 0.4) + (0.5 \times 0.1) = 3.25$ QALYs.

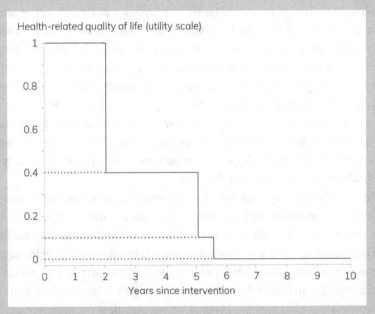

Figure 1 Quality-adjusted life years of a hypothetical patient

benefits over the relevant time horizon. These techniques are beyond the scope of this Element but have been explained in detail elsewhere.[67,68]

Figure 2 shows the possible combinations of incremental costs and benefits of a hypothetical improvement activity compared to the current status quo. If an activity falls into either cell A or D, then the adoption decision is straightforward. Activities in cell A offer greater benefits at a lower incremental cost than the alternative (status quo), and so should be adopted. An activity falling in cell D offers fewer health benefits at a higher cost than the alternative, and so should not be adopted.

The adoption decision for activities that fall into cells B and C is less clearcut, as there is a trade-off between benefits and costs. How can this trade-off be resolved? This requires assessing the opportunity cost of the adoption decision. The net effect of any activity can be quantified as the sum of two components: (1) the benefits of those who stand to benefit from the activity, and (2) the benefits that are lost elsewhere in the system (most likely by other people) because healthcare resources are diverted away to deliver the new activity. For example, having GPs work in hospital emergency departments to avoid non-urgent patients being admitted to the hospital takes them away from caring for patients in primary care settings.[69] If the net effect is positive, the activity generates more benefit than is sacrificed elsewhere; the activity thus offers value for money and should be adopted. If the net effect is negative, the intervention should not be adopted.

		Incremental benefits	
		Increase	Decrease
Incremental costs	Decrease	A	B
	Increase	C	D

Figure 2 Incremental costs and benefits of a hypothetical healthcare improvement activity relative to the status quo

In practice, the true opportunity costs of any healthcare improvement activity are rarely measured. There are two reasons for this. First, it is often not clear which existing healthcare activities would be defunded to release healthcare resources for the new activity. Second, even if those activities could be identified, their exact benefits are unlikely to be known because they have never been quantified formally.[70]

Most CEA applications therefore rely on approximations of the opportunity costs based on estimates of the amount of healthcare expenditure that is currently required to produce one unit of health (termed the 'marginal productivity' of the healthcare service). The most recent estimates for the English NHS put this figure at approximately £13,000 per QALY,[71] although previous figures of £30,000 per QALY are still widely used.

4.2 Evaluation in Action

To see the economic evaluation approach in action, we present three examples of CEAs of healthcare improvement activities in the English NHS. Each example focuses on an activity that promised to improve the provision of care, but in each case the value of the gains turned out to be lower than the benefits sacrificed if the activity was adopted. Nevertheless, two were implemented despite apparent lack of cost-effectiveness. This shows that CEA is just one criterion that decision-makers take into account when deciding what to implement.

4.2.1 Management of Multi-morbidity

Our first example focuses on efforts to improve the management of multi-morbidity in primary care. Clinical guidelines often emphasise a single-disease approach in which each disease is managed individually with limited regard for possible interactions between them.[72] This can lead to poorly coordinated and fragmented care pathways with suboptimal outcomes. The 3D (a mnemonic for 'dimensions of health, depression, and drugs') intervention sought to address this problem, taking a patient-centred approach to improving the care of patients with two or more long-standing illnesses.[73] It involves replacing annual, single-disease health checks with six-monthly 3D reviews that cover a patient's entire morbidity spectrum. Reviews are conducted by the patient's named GP together with a pharmacist and practice nurse. By taking a more holistic perspective, the 3D intervention is intended to improve continuity and coordination of care and to reduce the treatment burden for patients and carers.

The cost-effectiveness of the 3D intervention was evaluated in a cluster-randomised controlled trial involving 1,546 patients with multi-morbidity in 33 general practices in England and Scotland.[74] Practices were randomised to either the 3D intervention or usual care, and patients were followed up for 15 months. The trial identified a small but not statistically significant incremental health benefit of 0.007 QALYs per patient in the 3D intervention group. The incremental costs of the intervention were £126 per patient, which again was not statistically significantly different from zero. These incremental costs comprised the cost of delivering the intervention (e.g. staff training costs) as well as any changes in primary, secondary, and social care use, medication costs, and productivity losses (e.g. due to work absences) for patients and their carers as a result of the intervention. Given what we know about opportunity costs in the

English NHS, the 3D intervention is unlikely to be cost-effective. It would generate 0.007 QALYs per patient – but would require giving up 0.010 QALYs (= £126/£13,000 per QALY) per patient to fund the intervention.

It is possible that the reason the 3D intervention may not appear cost-effective is because of the relatively short follow-up period of the trial. Some of the benefits of changing the care arrangements for patients with complex multi-morbidity profiles might only arise at a later stage, whereas some of the costs only accrue once, at the beginning of the intervention. This demonstrates the need to conduct CEA over the full time period during which the consequences of an improvement activity could materialise. This would require using decision-analytic modelling to extrapolate information gained from randomised controlled trials that have limited follow-up periods.

4.2.2 Pay-for-performance

Our second example returns to the QOF, which is a characteristic example of a national pay-for-performance scheme of the type that economists see as important in sharpening the incentives for healthcare providers to improve (see Box 1). Since its introduction in 2004, discussions have continued about the scale and scope of the QOF and whether it remains fit for purpose. In 2016, the Scottish NHS abolished the QOF and redirected the money to GPs in the form of capitation payments instead.

To guide decision-making in other UK countries, Pandya et al.[75] compared the cost-effectiveness of two alternative strategies: (1) continue the QOF in its current form or (2) abolish it so that savings could be used to fund other NHS services. They focused on the costs and benefits of the QOF for patients aged 40–74 years with cardiovascular diseases and associated risk conditions (e.g. heart disease, stroke, diabetes, etc.), these accounting for the largest share of overall incentive payments made to GPs. The health benefits of the QOF were assessed by comparing mortality rates between the English NHS (where the QOF applied) and a selection of similar healthcare systems that did not have explicit financial incentives; on average, the QOF was associated with 58.9 fewer deaths per 100,000 population in those aged 40–74 with cardiovascular diseases.[75] These survival benefits were combined with information on HRQoL of individuals with cardiovascular diseases in order to calculate incremental lifetime QALYs for the general population. Additional health benefits (in the form of non-fatal events averted) were also calculated.

The incremental costs of the scheme considered in the analysis included: (1) the substantial incentive payments made to GP practices, (2) the direct costs of meeting the incentivised process standards (e.g. the cost of aspirin or other anticoagulants prescribed for patients with a history of chronic heart disease), as well as (3) any offsetting cost savings such as reductions in cardiovascular disease hospitalisations.

Overall, Pandya et al. report that the QOF did not generate sufficient health benefits to justify the costs of the scheme. At nearly £50,000 per QALY, the NHS had to give up more than three times as much health benefit to finance the QOF payments than it gained. This finding contradicts an earlier assessment of the QOF, which reached more favourable conclusions but was based on a less well-developed evidence base.[76] Although the reasons for the divergent findings are unclear, they highlight the need for continuous evaluation of healthcare improvement efforts as more evidence on their costs and benefits becomes available.

4.2.3 Comprehensive Hospital Emergency Services during Weekends

Our final example is a national healthcare improvement initiative aimed at improving emergency care in English NHS hospitals.[77] A number of studies have reported marked differences in risk-adjusted mortality between hospital patients admitted at weekends and those admitted during the week. This 'weekend mortality effect' has been linked to reduced levels of senior staffing and limited availability of diagnostic and support services on Saturdays and Sundays. In response to this suggestive evidence, English policymakers started to implement a comprehensive seven-day hospital service with constant staffing levels across all days of the week. These changes were predicted to cost the NHS between £1.07 billion and £1.43 billion per year in salaries and other expenditure. But was this the best use of money?

Meacock et al.[77] used CEA methods to inform the policy decision on the wider rollout of seven-day services in the English NHS. At the time their evaluation was conducted, the benefits of comprehensive seven-day services had not yet been established (they remain elusive even now). To overcome the lack of precise information, Meacock et al. set out to test whether the policy was likely to be cost-effective under different scenarios. The most optimistic scenario calculated the maximum potential health benefits of seven-day services by assuming that the policy would eliminate the excess weekend mortality rate of 0.35% (in 2011, mortality was 4.05% at weekends vs. 3.7% on weekdays); for England as a whole, this corresponded to approximately 4,400 excess deaths. These excess deaths in turn accounted for approximately 30,000 QALYs lost per year, calculated by quantifying the years of life lost and multiplying these with age-specific and sex-specific quality-of-life norms for the general population.

This suggested that comprehensive seven-day services had the potential to generate a large amount of health benefit for patients admitted at weekends. But in order to fund a seven-day service, the NHS would have to forgo approximately 82,300 QALYs (=£1.07 billion/£13,000 per QALY) in health benefits elsewhere in the system. So even under the most optimistic assumptions, the switch to a comprehensive seven-day service was highly unlikely to be a cost-effective use of limited NHS resources. This example illustrates that CEAs do not have to be complicated or use precise estimates of effectiveness to be informative. Fairly straightforward calculations can serve to establish bounds on the likely cost-effectiveness of healthcare improvement activities, reducing the need for more sophisticated evaluations.

5 Critiques of the Approach

Health economists have been influential in policy approaches to stimulate and evaluate improvements in healthcare, and they have had a major impact on healthcare systems in many countries. But there are critics of some of the approaches advocated by mainstream health economists.

Economists are not fully in consensus on the extent to which they believe that competition will foster improvements in healthcare. At one extreme, some argue that having governments involved in the healthcare system is not a panacea. They propose that people should instead be free to make their own decisions about their health and healthcare, free from government interference. These kinds of neoliberal views, which see 'government failure' as worse than 'market failure',[78,79] are commonly voiced in the USA, not just with respect to the healthcare system but for the economy in general.[80]

Neoliberalists, though, are in the minority among health economists. Most health economists recognise that healthcare systems are subject to market failure, most notably because of people's limited ability to assess their need for care and its quality and outcomes, as we discussed earlier. Indeed, Arrow's 1963 article[81] explaining these limitations is widely regarded as the seminal paper on which the sub-discipline of health economics was subsequently built.[82] The market failures that Arrow points to suggest that free markets with unbridled competition in the healthcare system are undesirable and justify government involvement to correct these market failures.

It is also important to be explicit that health economists are not blindly focused on saving money and do not advocate cost-cutting for the sake of it. Rather, they seek value for money, aiming to use resources as effectively and efficiently as possible. This is why health economists talk about opportunity costs, recognising that limited resources can be used in alternative ways. It is also why health economists have developed tools of economic evaluation, such as CEA, and argue that decision-makers need to take into account both costs and benefits when deciding how to make best use of the limited resources available to spend on healthcare. When health economists do propose reduced spending on a particular programme or activity, it is because it does not generate sufficient benefits to justify the expenditure, which could be used elsewhere to greater effect.

Finally, there is considerable debate among health economists about the objectives of the healthcare system and, therefore, the scale and scope of the evaluative space.[83] Some health economists argue that the ultimate aim of the healthcare system is (or ought to be) to maximise population health from the existing budget. This view has been highly influential in shaping how NICE (the National Institute for Health and Care Excellence) and similar agencies in other countries assess the cost-effectiveness of new medical technologies. Proponents of this approach can point to the QALY, which enables benefits to be summarised in a single, broad measure of health that facilitates comparisons of what is gained and what is forgone as a result of adoption decisions. Consequently, many CEAs conducted in the NHS focus on the QALY benefits that patients stand to gain or lose. But the focus on QALYs downplays or ignores other benefits, such as improved patient experience, timely access to care, and perhaps many of the other areas that are characteristically the focus of healthcare improvement activities.

The evidence that patients – and of course staff and other stakeholders – value so-called 'non-health' benefits in their own right is overwhelming.[83,84] This regularly leads to disagreements between various stakeholders about which activities offer value for money and which should be avoided. It is likely that calls to broaden the evaluative space beyond the QALY will ultimately be heeded, which implies adaption of the way that the opportunity costs of healthcare improvement activities are captured.

6 Further Research

There remain areas where further research is required, two of which are particularly pertinent to the preceding discussion. The first concerns whether economists have placed too much emphasis on competition as a driver of improvement in the healthcare sector and overlooked the possibility that improvements might come from people and organisations collaborating with each other. The second concerns how best to measure the benefits of health improvement activities, especially if these benefits extend beyond the healthcare sector.

6.1 Collaboration versus Competition

Health economists have traditionally focused on competition – but collaboration can be important in healthcare improvement too (see the Element on collaboration-based approaches[85]). A lot of empirical research has been undertaken to establish the impact of competition, usually relying on the assumption that organisations in close geographical proximity compete with one another. But organisations that are close to each other might actually collaborate, and this may be a good thing. For example, the reorganisation and centralisation of acute stroke services in London and in Manchester required service providers to work together to a common goal, thereby reducing competition between providers.[86] This model of collaboration brought about reductions in mortality and reductions in length of stay, yet clearly did not rely on market forces. Similar moves are underway to concentrate the provision of other services in specialist centres, particularly services for people with rare and complex conditions.[87]

As another example of collaboration, people living with multiple chronic conditions require care to be coordinated across healthcare settings and sometimes with other sectors also, notably social care. It is difficult to see how competition could ensure integrated care when responsibility is shared across multiple organisations. Collaboration rather than competition is much more likely to deliver benefits to those people.

A more accurate understanding of how healthcare organisations behave in terms of collaboration and competition is needed, as is a more precise measurement of these behaviours. In contributing to the evaluation of such activities, health economists need to question whether organisations in close proximity are in competition or are in fact collaborating. At present, the data used by economists means it is often difficult to tell collaboration and competition apart.

6.2 Economic Evaluation beyond Healthcare

Another important area for future research is how to extend the CEA framework to evaluate improvement activities that go beyond the scope of the healthcare system. CEA requires that benefits and opportunity costs can be expressed in the same metric, most commonly QALYs. This makes it possible to establish whether an intervention generates more benefits than are lost elsewhere. However, in many instances, at least some of the costs or benefits will fall outside the health sector. For example, improving implementation of alcohol misuse interventions could reduce future healthcare costs but could also influence the incidence of antisocial behaviour. The latter is of primary concern to the criminal justice system but has no direct relevance to the health service.

Should the health service fund an intervention that generates (perhaps mostly) non-health benefits in other areas of public service? And how should these benefits be accounted for in the CEA of healthcare improvement activities?

Steps are being taken towards answering such questions. Health economists have developed a general framework for conducting CEAs when the costs and benefits of interventions affect multiple sectors.[88,89] This framework emphasises the need to specify clearly for each sector (1) what outcome(s) they seek to maximise and (2) how productively they use their current budget to achieve this objective. Healthcare systems in many jurisdictions have taken clear positions on both issues, but other public services lag behind.[90] However, with an increasing emphasis on multi-sectoral collaborative working, the need to clarify these positions and to develop CEA methods that account for non-health benefits and opportunity costs is growing rapidly. This remains an evolving area of research and debate.

7 Conclusions

Economics is best described as a way of viewing the world, rather than a specific approach or methodology to improve healthcare. In this Element, we have applied economic thinking to examine how competitive pressures spur improvement, to identify how much competition and what inherent incentives healthcare organisations face to pursue improvements, and to explain the type of strategies that have been adopted to enhance those incentives. Economists have long argued that the healthcare market does not work well as a way of stimulating improvement, and their approach to healthcare improvement has therefore been to design policies that lower the opportunity costs of healthcare spending and improve the quality of services. These policies include regulation and inspection to assess quality, the introduction of competitive mechanisms to give service users more information and greater choice about where to receive care, payment arrangements designed to incentivise healthcare providers to become more efficient, and the tools of economic evaluation that allow comparison of the costs and benefits of using healthcare resources in alternative ways.

8 Further Reading

- Morris et al.[1] – an introductory textbook offering a UK focus and a balance of theory and applied analysis.
- Fuchs[91] – this book recognises the need to make choices at individual and societal levels in using scarce healthcare resources.

- Cookson et al.[92] – on the work of Alan Maynard, who was one of the world's most influential health economists. Maynard commented on subjects such as efficiency and equity, quality and outcomes, healthcare financing, markets, and competition.
- Drummond et al.[49,50] – now in its fourth edition, this is the go-to textbook for anyone required to undertake an economic evaluation.
- Briggs et al.[93] – a step-by-step guide to conducting an economic evaluation in Excel by some of the leading thinkers in this field.

Contributors

Andrew Street and Nils Gutacker contributed equally to the drafting of the Element and both authors have approved the final version.

Conflicts of Interest

Andrew Street and Nils Gutacker are both health economists.

Acknowledgements

We thank Simon Walker, the editors, and peer reviewers for their insightful comments and recommendations to improve the Element. A list of peer reviewers is published at www.cambridge.org/IQ-peer-reviewers.

Funding

This Element was funded by THIS Institute (The Healthcare Improvement Studies Institute, www.thisinstitute.cam.ac.uk). THIS Institute is strengthening the evidence base for improving the quality and safety of healthcare. THIS Institute is supported by a grant to the University of Cambridge from the Health Foundation – an independent charity committed to bringing about better health and healthcare for people in the UK.

About the Authors

Andrew Street is a professor of health economics with the London School of Economics and Political Science. He has worked for health departments in England and in Australia and has published numerous articles on topics including health system productivity, hospital efficiency, performance measurement, patient-reported outcomes, and integrated care.

Nils Gutacker is a professor of health economics with the University of York. His research focuses on the design and effectiveness of incentives, organisation of healthcare markets, unwarranted variation in healthcare provision, patient-reported outcome measures, and health inequalities.

Creative Commons License

References

1. Morris S, Devlin N, Parkin D, Spencer A. *Economic Analysis in Healthcare*. 2nd ed. John Wiley; 2012.
2. Newdick C. *Who Should We Treat? Rights, Rationing, and Resources in the NHS*. 2nd ed. Oxford: Oxford University Press; 2005. https://doi.org/10.1093/acprof:oso/9780199264186.001.0001.
3. Mason AR, Drummond MF. Public funding of new cancer drugs: Is NICE getting nastier? *Eur J Cancer* 2009; 45: 1188–92. https://doi.org/10.1016/j.ejca.2008.11.040.
4. Henderson J. The plastic surgery postcode lottery in England. *Int J Surg* 2009; 7: 550–8. https://doi.org/10.1016/j.ijsu.2009.09.004.
5. Shrank WH, Rogstad TL, Parekh N. Waste in the US health care system: Estimated costs and potential for savings. *JAMA* 2019; 322: 1501–9. https://doi.org/10.1001/jama.2019.13978.
6. Simoens S, De Coster S. Potential savings from increased substitution of generic for originator medicines in Europe. *J Generic Med* 2006; 4: 43–5. https://doi.org/10.1057/palgrave.jgm.4950040.
7. Popp W, Rasslan O, Unahalekhaka A, et al. What is the use? An international look at reuse of single-use medical devices. *Int J Hyg Environ Health* 2010; 213: 302–7. https://doi.org/10.1016/j.ijheh.2010.04.003.
8. Richardson G. Identifying, evaluating and implementing cost-effective skill mix. *J Nurs Manag* 1999; 7: 265–70. https://doi.org/10.1046/j.1365-2834.1999.00137.x.
9. Drucker PF. *Innovation and Entrepreneurship*. Oxford: Butterworth-Heinemann; 1985.
10. Care Quality Commission. *How We Monitor, Inspect and Regulate Adult Social Care Services*. www.cqc.org.uk/guidance-providers/adult-social-care/how-we-monitor-inspect-regulate-adult-social-care-services (accessed 1 March 2023).
11. NHS England. *GP Contract Documentation 2020/21*. www.england.nhs.uk/gp/investment/gp-contract/gp-contract-documentation-2020-21 (accessed 1 March 2023).
12. Roland M. Linking physicians' pay to the quality of care: A major experiment in the United Kingdom. *N Engl J Med* 2004; 351: 1448–54. https://doi.org/10.1056/NEJMhpr041294.
13. NHS England, NHS Improvement. *National Tariff Payment System: 2022/23*. www.england.nhs.uk/pay-syst/national-tariff/national-tariff-payment-system (accessed 1 March 2023).

14. Rodriguez Santana I, Mason A, Gutacker N, et al. Need, demand, supply in health care: Working definitions, and their implications for defining access. *Health Econ Policy Law* 2023; 18: 1–13. https://doi.org/10.1017/s1744133121 000293.

15. Mooney G, Ryan M. Agency in health care: Getting beyond first principles. *J Health Econ* 1993; 12: 125–35. https://doi.org/10.1016/0167-6296(93) 90023-8.

16. Rice T. The physician as the patient's agent. In: Jones A, ed. *The Elgar Companion to Health Economics*. 2nd ed. Cheltenham: Edward Elgar; 2013: 271–9.

17. James G. *Report of the Independent Inquiry into the Issues raised by Paterson*. London: HMSO; 2020. https://assets.publishing.service.gov.uk/government/ uploads/system/uploads/attachment_data/file/863211/issues-raised-by-pater son-independent-inquiry-report-web-accessible.pdf (accessed 19 May 2020).

18. Globerman S. *Select Cost Sharing in Universal Health Care Countries*. Vancouver, Canada: Fraser Institute; 2016. www.fraserinsti tute.org/studies/select-cost-sharing-in-universal-health-care-countries (accessed 1 March 2023).

19. Competition & Markets Authority. *Care Homes Market Study: Update Paper*. London: CMA; 2017. https://assets.publishing.service.gov.uk/ media/5941057be5274a5e4e00023b/care-homes-market-study-update-paper.pdf (accessed 19 May 2020).

20. LaingBuisson. *Care Homes for Older People UK Market Report*. 32nd ed. London: LaingBuisson; 2022. www.laingbuisson.com/shop/care-homes-for-older-people-uk-market-report-32ed (accessed 1 March 2023).

21. GOV.UK. *Attendance Allowance*. www.gov.uk/attendance-allowance#:~: text=change%20in%20circumstances-,Overview,need%20because%20of %20your%20disability (accessed 6 May 2021).

22. Forder J, Allan S. The impact of competition on quality and prices in the English care homes market. *J Health Econ* 2014; 34: 73–83. https://doi.org/ 10.1016/j.jhealeco.2013.11.010.

23. Allan S, Forder J. The determinants of care home closure. *Health Econ* 2015; 24: 132–45. https://doi.org/10.1002/hec.3149.

24. Matthews-King A. 'Alarming rise' in reports of care home abuse in England. *The Independent* (London); 23 June 2019. www.independent.co .uk/news/health/abuse-care-home-cqc-autism-learning-disability-whorl ton-hall-police-a8969026.html (accessed 1 March 2023).

25. NHS Digital. *Patients Registered at a GP Practice January 2020; Special Topic*. https://digital.nhs.uk/data-and-information/publications/ statistical/patients-registered-at-a-gp-practice/january-2020 (accessed 19 May 2020).

26. Santos R, Gravelle H, Propper C. Does quality affect patients' choice of doctor? Evidence from England. *Econ J* 2017; 127: 445–94. https://doi.org/10.1111/ecoj.12282.

27. Gravelle H, Liu D, Propper C, Santos R. Spatial competition and quality: Evidence from the English family doctor market. *J Health Econ* 2019; 68: 102249. https://doi.org/10.1016/j.jhealeco.2019.102249.

28. Nagraj S, Abel G, Paddison C, et al. Changing practice as a quality indicator for primary care: Analysis of data on voluntary disenrollment from the English GP Patient Survey. *BMC Fam Pract* 2013; 14: 89. https://doi.org/10.1186/1471-2296-14-89.

29. Stokes T, Dixon-Woods M, McKinley RK. Ending the doctor–patient relationship in general practice: A proposed model. *Fam Pract* 2004; 21: 507–14. https://doi.org/10.1093/fampra/cmh506.

30. Maynard A, Marinker M, Pereira-Gray D. The doctor, the patient, and their contract. III. Alternative contracts: Are they viable? *BMJ* 1986; 292: 1438–40. https://doi.org/10.1136/bmj.292.6533.1438.

31. Department of Health. *Working for Patients*. CM 555. London: HMSO; 1989.

32. Dusheiko M, Gravelle H, Jacobs R, Smith P. The effect of financial incentives on gatekeeping doctors: Evidence from a natural experiment. *J Health Econ* 2006; 25: 449–78. https://doi.org/10.1016/j.jhealeco.2005.08.001.

33. Moberly T, Stahl-Timmins W. QOF now accounts for less than 10% of GP practice income. *BMJ* 2019; 365: l1489. https://doi.org/10.1136/bmj.l1489.

34. Doran T, Kontopantelis E, Valderas JM, et al. Effect of financial incentives on incentivised and non-incentivised clinical activities: Longitudinal analysis of data from the UK Quality and Outcomes Framework. *BMJ* 2011; 342: d3590. https://doi.org/10.1136/bmj.d3590.

35. Doran T, Fullwood C, Kontopantelis E, Reeves D. Effect of financial incentives on inequalities in the delivery of primary clinical care in England: Analysis of clinical activity indicators for the quality and outcomes framework. *Lancet* 2008; 372: 728–36. https://doi.org/10.1016/S0140-6736(08)61123-X.

36. Forbes L, Marchand C, Peckham S. *Review of the Quality and Outcomes Framework in England: Final Report*. University of Kent: PRUComm; 2016. https://prucomm.ac.uk/assets/uploads/blog/2017/02/Review-of-QOF-21st-December-2016.pdf (accessed 6 May 2021).

37. Ryan AM, Krinsky S, Kontopantelis E, Doran T. Long-term evidence for the effect of pay-for-performance in primary care on mortality in the UK: A population study. *Lancet* 2016; 388: 268–74. https://doi.org/10.1016/S0140-6736(16)00276-2.

38. Checkland K, McDonald R, Harrison S. Ticking boxes and changing the social world: Data collection and the new UK general practice contract. *Soc Policy Admin* 2007; 41: 693–710. https://doi.org/10.1111/j.1467-9515.2007.00580.x.

39. Webster C. *The National Health Service: A Political History*. Oxford: Oxford University Press; 1998.

40. Busse R, Geissler A, Aaviksoo A, et al. Diagnosis related groups in Europe: Moving towards transparency, efficiency, and quality in hospitals? *BMJ* 2013; 346: f3197. https://doi.org/10.1136/bmj.f3197.

41. Grašič K, Mason A, Street A. Paying for the quantity and quality of hospital care: The foundations and evolution of payment policy in England. *Health Econ Rev* 2015; 5: 15. https://doi.org/10.1186/s13561-015-0050-x.

42. O'Reilly J, Busse R, Häkkinen U, et al. Paying for hospital care: The experience with implementing activity-based funding in five European countries. *Health Econ Policy Law* 2012; 7: 73–101. https://doi.org/10.1017/S1744133111000314.

43. NHS England. *Consultant Outcomes Publication*. www.england.nhs.uk/2014/11/outcome-publication (accessed 19 May 2020).

44. Healthcare Quality Improvement Partnership. *Clinical Outcomes Publication*. www.hqip.org.uk/national-programmes/clinical-outcomes-publication/#.Xj2SLmj7TIU (accessed 19 May 2020).

45. Bevan G, Hood C. What's measured is what matters: Targets and gaming in the English public health care system. *Public Admin* 2006; 84: 517–38. https://doi.org/10.1111/j.1467-9299.2006.00600.x.

46. NHS England, NHS Improvement. *National Tariff Payment System 2022/23. Annex C: Guidance on Best Practice Tariffs*. London: NHS England and NHS Improvement; 2022. www.england.nhs.uk/wp-content/uploads/2020/11/22-23NT_Annex-C-Best-practice-tariffs.pdf (accessed 1 March 2023).

47. McIlvennan CK, Eapen ZJ, Allen LA. Hospital readmissions reduction program. *Circulation* 2015; 131: 1796–803. https://doi.org/10.1161/CIRCULATIONAHA.114.010270.

48. Milstein R, Schreyoegg J. Pay for performance in the inpatient sector: A review of 34 P4P programs in 14 OECD countries. *Health Policy* 2016; 120: 1125–40. https://doi.org/10.1016/j.healthpol.2016.08.009.

49. Drummond M, McGuire A. *Economic Evaluation in Health Care: Merging Theory with Practice*. Oxford: Oxford University Press; 2001.

50. Drummond M, Sculpher M, Claxton K, Stoddart G, Torrance G. *Methods for the Economic Evaluation of Health Care Programmes*. 4th ed. Oxford: Oxford University Press; 2015.

51. Shah K, Praet C, Devlin N, et al. Is the aim of the English health care system to maximize QALYs? *J Health Serv Res Policy* 2012; 17: 157–63. https://doi.org/10.1258/jhsrp.2012.011098.

52. Williams A. The economic role of health indicators. In: Smith GT, ed. *Measuring the Social Benefit of Medicine*. London: Office of Health Economics; 1983: 63–7.

53. Lovibond K, Jowett S, Barton P, et al. Cost-effectiveness of options for the diagnosis of high blood pressure in primary care: A modelling study. *Lancet* 2011; 378: 1219–30. https://doi.org/10.1016/S0140-6736(11)61184-7.

54. Roze S, Isitt J, Smith-Palmer J, Javanbakht M, Lynch P. Long-term cost-effectiveness of Dexcom G6 real-time continuous glucose monitoring versus self-monitoring of blood glucose in patients with type 1 diabetes in the U.K. *Diabetes Care* 2020; 43: 2411–7. https://doi.org/10.2337/dc19-2213.

55. Stahl JE, Sandberg WS, Daily B, et al. Reorganizing patient care and workflow in the operating room: A cost-effectiveness study. *Surgery* 2006; 139: 717–28. https://doi.org/10.1016/j.surg.2005.12.006.

56. Wu RC, Laporte A, Ungar WJ. Cost-effectiveness of an electronic medication ordering and administration system in reducing adverse drug events. *J Eval Clin Pract* 2007; 13: 440–8. https://doi.org/10.1111/j.1365-2753.2006.00738.x.

57. Morris S, Ramsay AIG, Boaden RJ, et al. Impact and sustainability of centralising acute stroke services in English metropolitan areas: Retrospective analysis of hospital episode statistics and stroke national audit data. *BMJ* 2019; 364: ll. https://doi.org/10.1136/bmj.ll.

58. Basu A. Estimating costs and valuations of non-health benefits in cost-effectiveness analysis. In: Neumann PJ, Sanders GD, Russell LB, Siegel JE, Ganiats TG, eds. *Cost-effectiveness in Health and Medicine*. 2nd ed. Oxford: Oxford University Press; 2017: 201–36.

59. Basu A, Meltzer D. Implications of spillover effects within the family for medical cost-effectiveness analysis. *J Health Econ* 2005; 24: 751–73. https://doi.org/10.1016/j.jhealeco.2004.12.002.

60. Tubeuf S, Saloniki E-C, Cottrell D. Parental health spillover in cost-effectiveness analysis: Evidence from self-harming adolescents in England. *PharmacoEcon* 2019; 37: 513–30. https://doi.org/10.1007/s40273-018-0722-6.

62. Williams A. Economics of coronary artery bypass grafting. *BMJ* 1985; 291: 326–9. https://doi.org/10.1136/bmj.291.6491.326.

62. MacKillop E, Sheard S. Quantifying life: Understanding the history of quality-adjusted life-years (QALYs). *Soc Sci Med* 2018; 211: 359–66. https://doi.org/10.1016/j.socscimed.2018.07.004.

63. Prieto L, Sacristán JA. Problems and solutions in calculating quality-adjusted life years (QALYs). *Health Qual Life Outcomes* 2003; 1: 80. https://doi.org/10.1186/1477-7525-1-80.

64. Richardson J, Iezzi A, Khan MA. Why do multi-attribute utility instruments produce different utilities: The relative importance of the descriptive systems, scale and 'micro-utility' effects. *Qual Life Res* 2015; 24: 2045–53. https://doi.org/10.1007/s11136-015-0926-6.

65. Spiegelhalter D, Gore S, Fitzpatrick R, et al. Quality of life measures in health care. III: Resource allocation. *BMJ* 1992; 305: 1205–9. https://doi.org/10.1136/bmj.305.6863.1205.

66. Toulany A, Shojania K. Measurement for improvement. In: Dixon-Woods M, Brown K, Marjanovic S, et al., eds. *Elements of Improving Quality and Safety in Healthcare*. Cambridge: Cambridge University Press; forthcoming.

67. Briggs A, Sculpher M, Claxton K. *Decision Modelling for Health Economic Evaluation*. Oxford: Oxford University Press; 2006.

68. Gray AM, Clarke PM, Wolstenholme J, Wordsworth S. *Applied Methods of Cost-Effectiveness Analysis in Healthcare*. Oxford: Oxford University Press; 2010.

69. Gaughan J, Liu D, Gutacker N, et al. Does the presence of general practitioners in emergency departments affect quality and safety in English NHS hospitals? A retrospective observational study. *BMJ Open* 2022; 12: e055976. https://doi.org/10.1136/bmjopen-2021-055976.

70. Maynard A. The powers and pitfalls of payment for performance. *Health Econ* 2011; 21: 3–12. https://doi.org/10.1002/hec.1810.

71. Claxton K, Martin S, Soares M, et al. Methods for the estimation of the National Institute for Health and Care Excellence cost-effectiveness threshold. *Health Technol Assess* 2015; 19(14). https://doi.org/10.3310/hta19140.

72. Guthrie B, Payne K, Alderson P, McMurdo MET, Mercer SW. Adapting clinical guidelines to take account of multimorbidity. *BMJ* 2012; 345: e6341. https://doi.org/10.1136/bmj.e6341.

73. Salisbury C, Man M-S, Chaplin K, et al. A patient-centred intervention to improve the management of multimorbidity in general practice: The 3D RCT. *Health Serv Deliv Res* 2019; 7(5). https://doi.org/10.3310/hsdr07050.

74. Thorn J, Man M-S, Chaplin K, et al. Cost-effectiveness of a patient-centred approach to managing multimorbidity in primary care: A pragmatic cluster

randomised controlled trial. *BMJ Open* 2020; 10: e030110. https://doi.org/ 10.1136/bmjopen-2019-030110.

75. Pandya A, Doran T, Zhu J, et al. Modelling the cost-effectiveness of pay-for-performance in primary care in the UK. *BMC Med* 2018; 16: 135. https://doi.org/10.1186/s12916-018-1126-3.

76. Walker S, Mason AR, Claxton K, et al. Value for money and the Quality and Outcomes Framework in primary care in the UK NHS. *Br J Gen Pract* 2010; 60: e213–20. https://doi.org/10.3399/bjgp10X501859.

77. Meacock R, Doran T, Sutton M. What are the costs and benefits of providing comprehensive seven-day services for emergency hospital admissions? *Health Econ* 2015; 24: 907–12. https://doi.org/10.1002/hec.3207.

78. Le Grand J. The theory of government failure. *Br J Polit Sci* 1991; 21: 423–42. https://doi.org/10.1017/S0007123400006244.

79. Wolf C. *Markets or Governments: Choosing between Imperfect Alternatives.* 2nd ed. Cambridge, MA: MIT Press; 1993.

80. Klein N. *The Shock Doctrine.* London: Penguin; 2008.

81. Arrow KJ. Uncertainty and the welfare economics of medical care. *Am Econ Rev* 1963; 53: 941–73. www.jstor.org/stable/1812044 (accessed 1 March 2023).

82. Fuchs V. Kenneth Arrow's legacy and the article that launched a thousand studies. *Health Affairs*; 8 March 2017. https://doi.org/10.1377/forefront .20170308.059100.

83. Hansen P. Health sector decision-making: More than just cost per QALY calculations. *J Health Serv Res Policy* 2012; 17: 129–30. https://doi.org/ 10.1258/JHSRP.2012.012058.

84. Ryan M, Gerard K. Inclusiveness in the health economic evaluation space. *Soc Sci Med* 2014; 108: 248–51. https://doi.org/10.1016/j.socscimed.2014.01.035.

85. Martin G, Dixon-Woods M. Collaboration-based approaches. In: Dixon-Woods M, Brown K, Marjanovic S, et al., eds. *Elements of Improving Quality and Safety in Healthcare.* Cambridge: Cambridge University Press; 2022. https://doi.org/10.1017/9781009236867.

86. Morris S, Hunter RM, Ramsay AIG, et al. Impact of centralising acute stroke services in English metropolitan areas on mortality and length of hospital stay: Difference-in-differences analysis. *BMJ* 2014; 349: g4757. https://doi.org/10.1136/bmj.g4757.

87. Bojke C, Grašič K, Street A. How should hospital reimbursement be refined to support concentration of complex care services? *Health Econ* 2018; 27: e26–38. https://doi.org/10.1002/hec.3525.

88. Walker S, Griffin S, Asaria M, Tsuchiya A, Sculpher M. Striving for a societal perspective: A framework for economic evaluations when costs

and effects fall on multiple sectors and decision makers. *Appl Health Econ Health Policy* 2019; 17: 577–90. https://doi.org/10.1007/s40258-019-00481-8.

89. Ramponi F, Walker S, Griffin S, et al. Cost-effectiveness analysis of public health interventions with impacts on health and criminal justice: An applied cross-sectoral analysis of an alcohol misuse intervention. *Health Econ* 2021; 30: 972–88. https://doi.org/10.1002/hec.4229.

90. Hinde S, Walker SM, Lortie-Forgues H. *Applying the Three Core Concepts of Economic Evaluation in Health to Education in the UK*. Discussion Paper. CHE Research Paper. York: Centre for Health Economics, University of York; 2019. https://eprints.whiterose.ac.uk/153488 (accessed 1 March 2023).

91. Fuchs VR. *Who Shall Live? Health, Economics and Social Choice.* 2nd ed. Singapore: World Scientific; 2011. https://doi.org/10.1142/8167.

92. Cookson R, Goddard M, Sheldon T, eds. *Maynard Matters: Critical Thinking on Health Policy.* York: YPS; 2016.

93. Briggs A, Sculpher M, Claxton K. *Decision Modelling for Health Economic Evaluation.* Oxford: Oxford University Press; 2006.

Cambridge Elements ☰

Improving Quality and Safety in Healthcare

Editors-in-Chief

Mary Dixon-Woods
THIS Institute (The Healthcare Improvement Studies Institute)

Mary is Director of THIS Institute and is the Health Foundation Professor of Healthcare Improvement Studies in the Department of Public Health and Primary Care at the University of Cambridge. Mary leads a programme of research focused on healthcare improvement, healthcare ethics, and methodological innovation in studying healthcare.

Graham Martin
THIS Institute (The Healthcare Improvement Studies Institute)

Graham is Director of Research at THIS Institute, leading applied research programmes and contributing to the institute's strategy and development. His research interests are in the organisation and delivery of healthcare, and particularly the role of professionals, managers, and patients and the public in efforts at organisational change.

Executive Editor

Katrina Brown
THIS Institute (The Healthcare Improvement Studies Institute)

Katrina is Communications Manager at THIS Institute, providing editorial expertise to maximise the impact of THIS Institute's research findings. She managed the project to produce the series.

Editorial Team

Sonja Marjanovic
RAND Europe

Sonja is Director of RAND Europe's healthcare innovation, industry, and policy research. Her work provides decision-makers with evidence and insights to support innovation and improvement in healthcare systems, and to support the translation of innovation into societal benefits for healthcare services and population health.

Tom Ling
RAND Europe

Tom is Head of Evaluation at RAND Europe and President of the European Evaluation Society, leading evaluations and applied research focused on the key challenges facing health services. His current health portfolio includes evaluations of the innovation landscape, quality improvement, communities of practice, patient flow, and service transformation.

Ellen Perry
THIS Institute (The Healthcare Improvement Studies Institute)

Ellen supported the production of the series during 2020–21.

About the Series

The past decade has seen enormous growth in both activity and research on improvement in healthcare. This series offers a comprehensive and authoritative set of overviews of the different improvement approaches available, exploring the thinking behind them, examining evidence for each approach, and identifying areas of debate.

Cambridge Elements ≡

Improving Quality and Safety in Healthcare

Elements in the Series

Collaboration-Based Approaches
Graham Martin and Mary Dixon-Woods

Co-Producing and Co-Designing
Glenn Robert, Louise Locock, Oli Williams, Jocelyn Cornwell, Sara Donetto, and Joanna Goodrich

The Positive Deviance Approach
Ruth Baxter and Rebecca Lawton

Implementation Science
Paul Wilson and Roman Kislov

Making Culture Change Happen
Russell Mannion

Operational Research Approaches
Martin Utley, Sonya Crowe, and Christina Pagel

Reducing Overuse
Caroline Cupit, Carolyn Tarrant, and Natalie Armstrong

Simulation as an Improvement Technique
Victoria Brazil, Eve Purdy, and Komal Bajaj

Workplace Conditions
Jill Maben, Jane Ball, and Amy C. Edmondson

Governance and Leadership
Naomi J. Fulop and Angus I. G. Ramsay

Health Economics
Andrew Street and Nils Gutacker

A full series listing is available at: www.cambridge.org/IQ.

Printed in the United States
by Baker & Taylor Publisher Services

Printed in the United States
by Baker & Taylor Publisher Services